SUCCESS
with
Potty Training!

SUCCESS
with
Potty Training!

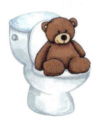

Teach and model before taking the diaper off your toddler for clean, fast results!

Beth Allen

Copyright © 2023 by Beth Allen.

All rights reserved. No part of this book may be used or reproduced in any form whatsoever without written permission except in the case of brief quotations in critical articles or reviews.

Printed in the United States of America.

For more information, or to book an event, contact:
http://www.successwithpottytraining.com
Beth@successwithpottytraining.com

ISBN - Paperback: 979-8-9870264-1-0
First Edition: January 2023

This publication contains the opinions and ideas of its author. It is intended to provide helpful and informative material on the subjects addressed in the publication. It is sold with the understanding that the author and publisher are not engaged in rendering medical, health, or any other kind of personal professional services in the book. The reader should consult their medical, health, or other competent professional before adopting any of the suggestions in this book or drawing inferences from it.

Table of Contents

Chapter 1: The Problem 1

Chapter 2: The Real Goal and Your Role as the Coach 7

Chapter 3: A Focused, and Motivated Child 15

Chapter 4: Is My Child Ready? 21

Pre-Assessment Checklist 29

Chapter 5: Supplies 31

Supplies Quick List 32

Chapter 6: Getting a Little Bum on a Big Toilet 33

Chapter 7: Here We Go! I'll Take You Step-by-Step 37

    Step #1 Teach and Model 38

    Step #2 Motivate 42

    Step #3 Helping A Lot! 43

Chapter 8: Step #4 Problem Solve 51

    The Three Types of Problems 51

    Problem #1: Understanding 51

    Problem #2: Motivational 55

    Problem #3: Behavioral 56

Chapter 9: Accidents 63

Chapter 10: Training for Naps and Night 67

Chapter 11: It's All You Kid 73

    Taking a Break 74

Chapter 12: The Scoop on Poop	77
Chapter 13: More Help!	81
First Time Out of the House	81
Car Trips	81
Tips	82
Proper Wiping	83
FAQs	83
Chapter 14: I Have to Go to Work!	87
A Small Ask	89
Plan Outline	90
Bathroom Steps Chart	92
Index	95
References	98

Chapter 1: The Problem

You really need your child out of diapers!

It puts a pit in your stomach to think about having to clean up pee and poop. I get it. The thought of potty training a child can make anyone nervous, but you need to stop spending your hard-earned money on diapers. You don't want to keep changing them; they're gross. You're feeling the social pressure of your child getting older, but where do you start? You've heard horror stories, and now you're nervous. You don't want those horror stories to be you. No, you need to be the one whose child caught on so quickly that it only took one weekend, and it was no big deal.

There's a lot at risk if your child doesn't seem to catch on quickly. Nobody wants to continuously clean up accidents.

I was with a friend when I noticed her son was in a pull-up. Being the certified potty training consultant I am, I asked her about it. She looked sick when she told me about her first attempt at potty training. She had followed another method, and it had gone south quickly. She said when she took the diaper off her son, he started peeing everywhere. He didn't seem to get it. Not knowing what to do to get him to stop having accidents, she threw up her hands and put him in a pull-up. That's where I came in. I told her I believe you should explain using the bathroom to your child before taking off their diaper. Teach and model the concept first, so your child has a chance to understand what's going on.

I told her I want my child to pee like me, meaning, in the bathroom, with a real toilet, in actual underwear, using all the same bathroom steps I do. This was so much more logical to her. Of course, that's what she wanted for her son too. She signed up for a consultation session. I taught her my method, and after only a few days, I got a text from her. Here's what it read:

> *Beth, this really has been a game changer for us! We just put him down for bed (in underwear), and he officially had zero accidents today! We're so happy and amazed at how well he has done these past few days. We can't thank you enough for sharing your method with us!*

The nervous pit in my friend's stomach had turned to joy!

I am so excited to share with you this revolutionary approach to potty training. Potty training is tough. There are a lot of obstacles to overcome. What I'm about to share with you will be life changing. When a parent potty trains their child,

Chapter 1: The Problem

it's a huge growing moment for both the parent and their child.

Why is this method revolutionary? Lately, the potty training methods have really digressed. When I potty trained my first child, I read up on all the methods, and watched all the latest videos. I felt prepared, but I failed miserably. It was hard to take. Like most moms who fail at potty training, I blamed myself and my ability to be a "good mom." Then, I blamed my child and thought maybe there was a problem. Never once did I think to blame the method.

I then had some eye-opening experiences. These experiences helped me recognize the shortcomings of these methods. My son suffered from chronic ear infections. These ear infections caused my son to temporarily lose his hearing. Though my son is very intelligent, losing his hearing resulted in him having a hard time with speech. I was able to have professionals come into my home through early intervention programs and help with speech delays. These women were amazing! With their professional training, they were able to work with my son on his speech, introducing us to Play-Based Learning.

Play-Based Learning was fascinating to me. The professionals would sit on the floor with toys. They would use the toys to model a task they'd like my son to do. They would demonstrate the task, and then they would help my son copy the demonstration. I sat transfixed, watching my son's reaction to their teaching.

These professionals were so purposeful in their play. It was very articulated and prepared. I loved the idea of teaching through play. When a child is playing while learning, they're so motivated. They progress so quickly.

My son was captivated. He learned and progressed, all while thinking he was just playing and having a good time. I studied their methods, and it dawned on me that the reason I had failed at potty training was not because of my abilities, or my son's abilities, but because the methods I had tried were flawed. I realized I needed a method that modeled the behavior I wanted my son to achieve from potty training.

It energized me to discover a new way to teach my child. This gave me the motivation to create a new potty training method. My new method was a hit! My next three children all potty trained in a day or two. Now, as a certified potty training consultant, (yes, that's a real thing) others I have trained in my method have also trained in just a couple of days.

I'm excited to help you realize the real goals of potty training. I'm excited to teach you how to get a focused and motivated child with Play-Based Learning and modeling. In this book, I'll introduce you to the famous child psychologist, Lev Vygotsky, and how he taught that we should properly set up scaffolding around your child so you can assist them correctly toward success. I'm not saying your child will train in a day, but you will be impressed with the amount of progress you see in a short amount of time.

You'll have more money in your pocket, and a smile on your face because your child is now in underwear, and it was no big deal.

It's those who have gone about this the wrong way who turn this great milestone into a time of frustration and agony. Do this wrong, and it becomes a wedge driven between you and your child.

Following this method will give you freedom from diapers. It will give you and your child a sense of accomplishment and will form the kind of bond any good coach has with their successful team.

So, let's do this the right way! The professional way, the way that works! You've got this!

Chapter 2: The Real Goal and Your Role as the Coach

Many parents unknowingly go into potty training with the wrong goal in mind. They think the goal is to see how many times their child can pee in the toilet. This leads to actions such as a sticker on a chart for every time their child pees, or having their child drink tons of juice to get them to pee more, or spending all day in the bathroom with your child just sitting on the toilet waiting to see if they can pee again. Even worse, many methods have your child pee in a little potty chair. They encourage you to place the potty chair anywhere in the house with your child peeing in the playroom, living room, kitchen, and so on. These actions cause confusion and exhaustion with your child. They ultimately lead to resistance and rebellion. These actions will not get you to your real goal. So, let's take a minute to make sure we know why we're potty training, and what the real goal is. First, here are the reasons to potty train:

- You need your child to take care of their own hygiene needs.
- You want to stop using and changing diapers.
- You want your child to wear underwear and keep their underwear clean and dry.
- You want all the pee and poop to be in the toilet.
- You want your child to do this independently, letting you know if they need help.

I cannot emphasize enough how important it is to use the actual toilet. This will help set the household-wide expectation that everyone in the house only pees and poops in the toilet, in the bathroom. This will be reinforced every time they see someone else go into the bathroom. This will avoid any confusion about what the expectation is.

The Real Goal

Now for the real goal of potty training. The goal is for your child to take care of their own hygiene needs. They do this by wearing underwear instead of diapers, keeping that underwear clean and dry by peeing and pooping in the toilet, and adequately following all the bathroom steps.

The goal should be explained to your child in the following words: "You need to keep your underwear clean and dry. I am here to help you! Tell me if the pee is coming so I can help you keep your underwear clean and dry by going to the bathroom."

After realizing the goal, it seems natural that:

1. The child needs to at least be wearing underwear while training. Pants, skirts, and shorts that are easy to pull up and down are also okay.
2. While training, your child needs to be using the same toilet that you use. (An actual toilet, not a small potty one.)

3. You will focus on keeping their underwear clean and dry, instead of focusing on how many times they pee.
4. Rewards will be earned when the child uses the bathroom as well as other areas of focus. You will use rewards to encourage progression throughout the process.

Remember, it is not your goal to make your child hold their pee while running around naked. Moreover, it is not the goal of this training to make your child pee in a miniature potty, peeing and pooping anywhere in the house they please. Keep in mind what you actually want out of this, and what it is you're trying to accomplish.

So, I'll restate the goal. The goal is for your child to take care of their own hygiene needs. They do this by wearing underwear instead of diapers, keeping that underwear clean and dry by peeing and pooping in the toilet, and adequately following all the bathroom steps.

Success With Potty Training

The Coach

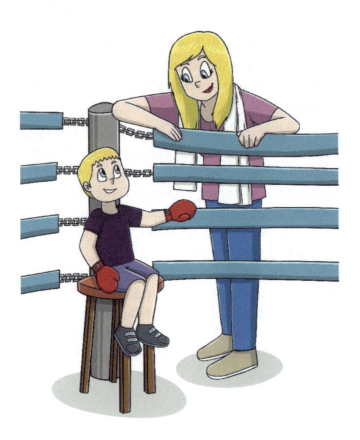

As potty training starts, it is tempting to have the mindset of You vs. Your Child, but this mindset is incorrect. You're the coach; you're on the same team. This isn't you against your child. This isn't you forcing your child.

Picture a child inside a boxing ring. You are not in the ring, boxing it out with your child. You are not your child's opponent. Instead, the child is in the ring, boxing it out with the *unwanted behavior*, in this case, using a diaper.

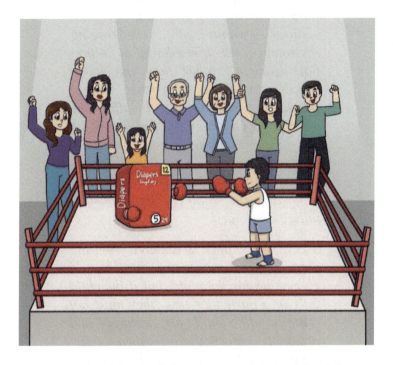

You are the *coach*. You are on the *outside* of the ring; you remain the calm, professional, more knowledgeable adult. You are going to help your child knock out this old behavior.

Ultimately, the child is taking responsibility for achieving this new milestone. It is the child who is in the game. You are there to help them understand what the process and expectations are, and the steps they will take to succeed. You will help them learn the new skills and rules. You're there to help coach them through the process. Erik Erikson, a child developmental psychologist, stated:

> *It is critical that parents allow their children to explore the limits of their abilities within an encouraging environment which is tolerant of failure. For example, rather than put on a child's clothes, a supportive parent should have the patience to allow the child to try until they succeed or ask for assistance. So, the parents need to encourage the child to become more independent while at the same time protecting the child so that constant failure is avoided.*
>
> *A delicate balance is required from the parent. They must try not to do everything for the child, but if the child fails at a particular task, they must not criticize the child for failures and accidents (particularly when toilet training). The aim has to be "Self-control without a loss of self-esteem" (Gross, 1992).*[1]

---

[1] Dr. Saul McLeod, "Erik Erikson's Stages of Psychosocial Development," Simply Psychology, 2018, https://www.simplypsychology.org/Erik-Erikson.html

Chapter 2: The Real Goal and Your Role as the Coach

As the child learns and tries, you calmly coach correction, give reinforcement, restate the goal, and give motivation. As a coach, you'll need to repeat instructions and keep the end goal in mind. Let your child know you're there to help, and if they tell you when they need to go, then you'll be right there to help them. You're a positive, inspiring coach, and you've got this!

Chapter 3: A Focused, and Motivated Child

To shorten the time it takes to potty train, we need a focused, motivated, and persistent child. We need a child who understands what we're doing and wants it just as much as we do. So how do we do this? Is this some magic? No, well maybe, it's called Play-Based Learning, modeling, and scaffolding, and it works!

Play-Based Learning and Modeling

Think of a time when your child was playing with a new toy. They're fascinated with it. It only takes a little guidance and prompting from you, and then you can leave them with it, and they'll persist in trying all kinds of new things. They are much more focused and receptive to learning during play. Playing captivates their attention, motivates, stimulates, and supports their development of skills.

When we start out by playing, we break down barriers. We are creating an environment that is fun and safe. This immediately relieves the child of any pressure. It's ok to try new things when you're playing. Children are more willing to persist in learning something new or solving a problem while playing.

We want potty training to be accomplished in the shortest amount of time. When a child is involved in Play-Based Learning, they are much more likely to be focused, motivated, and persistent. This allows us to teach them more efficiently.

A playing child is also determined and empowered to take ownership and responsibility for their own learning.[2] The ultimate goal is to have the child take responsibility for their own hygiene needs. We want the child to feel ownership in this process, and there's no better way than play. The sooner they take responsibility, the better.

Play-Based Learning is not silly time, though. It is carefully articulated and planned out. You are the facilitator. The toys become coaching and teaching tools. The child is having fun, but is being thoughtfully guided by you. Children do much of their learning through pretend play and role-playing.[3] We will capitalize on this by allowing them to role-play the training method first with a teddy bear.

Using a teddy bear will engage the child's attention. Modeling the bathroom steps with the teddy bear will allow them to fully see what is expected, what the new rules are, and what the reward is. Having the child understand all of this avoids initial power struggles and confusion.

---

[2] "What is Play-Based Learning," Government of Northwest Territories, January 2017, Retrieved From: https://www.ece.gov.nt.ca/sites/ece/files/resources/fact_sheet_-_play_based_learning_en.pdf.

[3] Dr. Saul McLeod, "The Preparational Stage of Cognitive Development," Simply Psychology, 2018, https://www.simplypsychology.org/preoperational.html

Scaffolding

Lev Vygotsky, known for his work on psychological development in children, said, "What a child can do in cooperation today, he can do alone tomorrow." He taught that in order for a child to be able to do tasks, they must first be guided by a more knowledgeable other. Vygotsky refers to this guidance as scaffolding. Though scaffolding is used in various ways he describes scaffolding as being supportive. With the scaffolding up, the building is able to be worked on. As the building is gradually able to hold its own, the scaffolding is taken down. Vygotsky described this scaffolding process with a child as such:

- Getting ready: Gaining and maintaining the learner's interest in the task.
- Show me how: Demonstrating the task.
- Help me do it: Making the task simple. Getting down on their level.
- Controlling the child's level of frustration. (Looking for triggers.)
- Let me do it myself: Emphasizing certain aspects that will help with the solution. [4]

---

[4] Dr. Saul McLeod, "The Zone of Proximal Development and Scaffolding", Simply Psychology, 2019, https://www.simplypsychology.org/Zone-of-Proximal-Development.html

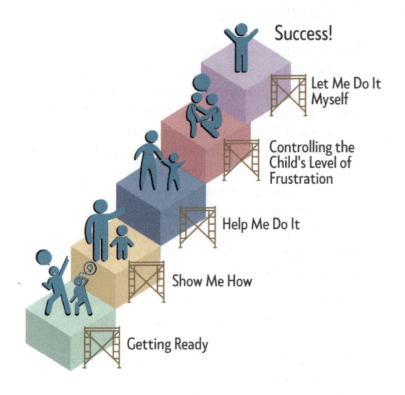

Here's how we apply Vygotsky's scaffolding to our potty training: You'll first captivate their attention by modeling how to properly use the toilet with a teddy bear. You'll demonstrate how to use the bathroom by breaking down the steps, making them simple and on their level. You'll be with them, adjusting your support to meet their abilities, allowing them to do as much as possible on their own, all while controlling the frustration level.

Your assistance to your child will be most effective when you vary your help according to how your child is doing. When your child is doing well, become less specific with your help. When your child starts to struggle, give increasingly more specific instructions until your child starts to make progress again.[5][6]

With the excitement of Play-Based Learning, modeling the expectations, and the assistance you provide through scaffolding, potty training will be a positive success for both you and your child. It will be an opportunity for them to accomplish something big and feel a sense of pride. It will allow you to show your child you're there to help them, and that together you can do this!

---

[5] Wood, D., Bruner, J., & Ross, G. (1976). "The role of tutoring in problem-solving." *Journal of Child Psychology and Child Psychiatry*, 17, 89–100.

[6] Wood, D., & Middleton, D. (1975). "A study of assisted problem-solving." *British Journal of Psychology*, 66(2), 181–191.

Chapter 4: Is My Child Ready?

I do not pick a certain age for a child to start potty training, but I will tell you some developmental milestones to look for that will help you determine when to start for your child. These milestones help make potty training successful.

First Assessment: Communicating Their Needs

The child needs to be able to communicate that they need to use the bathroom. Preferably this is done verbally. For example, "Mom, I need to use the bathroom," or just saying one word, like "potty" or "pee." This can also be nonverbal, such as holding their crotch while tugging on your shirt. It is crucial that your child can *intentionally communicate* their need to go to the bathroom, and that you're not the only one who will understand them. This way, you'll be able to leave them with their grandma, a babysitter, or at daycare. The way you assess this milestone is to see if they can communicate other things. For example, can they ask for a drink or ask you to pick them up? Can they tell you they want their diaper changed? If the answer is yes, this means they can communicate their needs.

Second Assessment: Following Simple Instructions

The child needs to be able to follow simple two-step instructions. For instance, can you tell them to go into the other room and get their shoes? Do they understand this expectation?

Third Assessment: Pulling Pants Down and Up

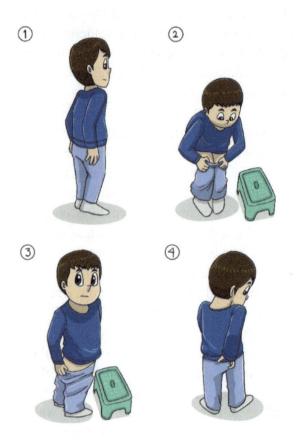

1. Reaching toward the back to pull down pants.
2. Pulling up pants to the knees.
3. Reaching to the middle of the back to pull pants over the bum.
4. Pulling up the middle of the back of the pants over the bum.

Your child needs to at least be able to pull their pants down. It would be ideal if they could pull down *and* pull up their pants. (You can decide if you want to be the one putting their pants back on for them each time they use the bathroom.) I highly recommend teaching this skill in advance. Practice with your child each day when they get dressed. Practicing beforehand will also let you know what clothes will be best for them to wear while potty training.

Pulling Down Pants: It's important for your child to get their pants down quickly. When a child decides they need to use the bathroom, they usually don't give themselves very much time. So, they can't be wrestling with their pants, or they'll end up peeing all over the floor. It's much quicker if you teach your child to reach slightly behind their hips to pull their pants down, this will help them get the elastic over their bum. Getting the pants over the hump of the bum is the hardest.

Pulling Up Pants: Have your child pull up their pants over their knees to get started. Then help them reach their hand to the middle of their back to help get the elastic over the bum. If they only pull up from the sides or front of the pants, then the pants will get stuck on their bum. So, have them reach behind to the middle of the back of the pants, and then pull up over the bum. This is a challenging skill for them and should not be learned the same day as potty training.

Fourth Assessment: Sitting Independently

Your child needs to be able to sit up in a chair on their own, so they'll be able to sit on the toilet on their own. So many times, we strap our children into seats, causing them to not have had the opportunity to sit independently.

Fifth Assessment: No Crib

The child cannot be sleeping in a confining crib, or a locked or gated room at night. They need to be able to get up first thing in the morning to use the bathroom.

Sixth Assessment: No Drinks in Bed

The child can't be going to bed with a bottle or large sippy cup in hand. They'll need to be weaned off having any liquids in bed with them. Liquids will need to be limited after dinner and before bed to help make night training successful. A small drink before bed is fine. If you've been using a cup as a soothing tool for your child to sleep, consider replacing it with reading them a book or singing them a lullaby.

Seventh Assessment: Diapers are Yucky

Start labeling dirty diapers as yucky. Start pointing out they don't want poop and pee on their bum.

Eighth Assessment: Bladder Control

See if your child can go for some time with a clean diaper. Make sure they're not just dribbling out pee all day, but that they pee in large amounts with times of dryness in-between. This will help ensure the bladder has developed enough to hold pee for some time in-between using the bathroom. It's typical for a two-year-old to be able to go two hours in-between peeing.

Ninth Assessment: Walking and Climbing

Your child will need to get themselves to the bathroom and then be able to climb up on a stool and get themselves onto the toilet. You can practice this skill by having them use a stool to climb up onto a chair. Or, go ahead and let them practice climbing up onto the toilet.

Tenth Assessment: Your Child's Understanding

Do you know if your child does or doesn't understand you? Start paying attention when you give your child instructions. Begin to establish good communication between you and your child. Try filling in the blanks:

My child communicates that they understand me by
_____.
(Nodding, looking at me, following the instruction, verbally saying ok, or repeating what I say, etc.)

My child communicates that they don't understand me by
_____.
(Ignoring me, staring blankly, throwing a fit, etc.)

Eleventh Assessment: Health

Is your child in good health? It's very hard to learn something new when you're sick. Your child should not be on medications that affect your child's bowel movements or sleeping patterns. Your child needs to be learning how it feels when they need to use the bathroom and should not be on large amounts of laxatives. Laxatives can make it very hard for your child to make it on time to the bathroom. Also, if your child is on medication that makes them sleepy, then it will be too difficult for them to get up in time to use the bathroom at night. If your pediatrician has recommended laxatives, you should talk with them to create a plan for what to do for potty training.

Twelfth Assessment: Fears

It's good to look at the bathroom steps and see if your child has any fears associated with any of them. Have your child try some of the steps. When getting ready for a bath, for instance, ask if they'd like to try sitting on the toilet. Sit them there for a second, and then take them right off. Praise them for trying and see what their reaction is. If they're scared, then you'll know they need to work on that ahead of time.

See if they'd like to flush the toilet. See how they react to the sound. Have them wash their hands in the bathroom. Start early by trying out a few of the steps so you can gauge their reaction.

Other helpful assessments to look for but not deal-breakers:

Pay attention at naptime and in the morning, to see if they wake up with a dry diaper. This isn't a must, but it is really helpful if you already know they can do this. A lot of times, kids will start waking up dry and then pee really soon afterwards, so check right when they wake up. If they have peed, but it's still warm, then that means they just did it. Praise them when they wake up dry.

See if your child has any desire to use the bathroom. If they've seen older siblings, or even you, use the bathroom a lot of times, they will be curious. If so, go ahead and help them sit on the toilet a few times and see their reaction. Start letting them into the bathroom and go ahead and point out the toilet. You can even let them flush it and use the sink to wash their hands. Learning any of the steps ahead of time will help shorten the actual potty training time.

Start pointing out underwear, for example, "Look, your cousin is now a big kid wearing undies." or "Do you see your brother's underwear? You can have underwear too if you want." or "Your friend John is now wearing underwear, he's a big kid. Wow! Way to go, John!" Start planting the seed of desire. Make sure this is positive and not in any way shaming your child.

You will need to set aside at least two days where you can expect to pay all your attention to your child and not go anywhere or need to do anything else. It's also helpful if the next couple of days after that are easy-going and flexible.

Things to Avoid

- Don't train right before moving to a new home.
- Don't train just before a big event, such as a wedding or the first day of daycare.
- Don't train right before your due date for another child.
- Don't train while you or your child is sick. Make sure everyone is well. Sickness makes learning something new too hard, and if you're sick, it's hard to have patience.
- Don't train if you'll be immediately taking a trip after day three or do anything too unusual or out of the normal schedule for a little while.

Pre-Assessment Checklist

See the chapter for more details.

My Child:
- ☐ Communicates their needs
- ☐ Follows simple instructions
- ☐ Sits independently
- ☐ Can pull down and up pants
- ☐ No crib or confined bedroom situation
- ☐ Weaned off any liquids in bed
- ☐ Has been prepped that diapers are yucky
- ☐ Has dry spells in-between dirty diapers
- ☐ Can walk and climb
- ☐ My child communicates they understand me by _____.
- ☐ My child communicates they don't understand me by _____.
- ☐ In good health
- ☐ I have addressed Fears

Chapter 5: Supplies

I don't believe you need any special potty chairs or accessories. Here's what you will need, though:

- 10 - 15 pairs of underwear that are one size too big, so the child can easily pull them up and down. Have fun with this; let your child pick them out. They can pick their favorite character or color.

- Pants, shorts, or skirts that are easy to pull down. They can't be too tight. Just elastic bands, no zippers, snaps, belts, onesies, or buttons. (Basketball shorts or sweatpants are a good option.)

- A large teddy bear, one that can wear the child's underwear.

- Treats or rewards, mix and match. A small treat you can give your child for each step, like mini marshmallows, skittles, or M&Ms, and then a larger treat for when they poop, like large marshmallows or mini candy bars. Some kids get tired of the same treat, if this is your child, then you might consider a treasure box for rewards. This can include stickers and other little rewards.

- Two waterproof mattress protectors for their bed and an extra sheet. If the mattress is already waterproof, then you'll just need the sheets.

- A step stool or two. One for the toilet and one for the sink.

- A bathroom steps chart for the bathroom. Cut out the one at the end of this book, or download one for free from my website www.successwithpottytraining.com.

- A nightlight for the bathroom, maybe one for the hallway as well.

- Indoor activities to play with (so you don't go stir crazy) such as play dough, coloring books, or cars.

- Cleaning supplies to clean up accidents, disinfectant wipes, and carpet cleaner, if you have carpet.

Supplies Quick List

See the back of the book for a list you can cut out.
- ☐ Underwear
- ☐ Easy clothes
- ☐ Teddy bear
- ☐ Treats or rewards (treasure box)
- ☐ Waterproof Mattress Protectors (2)
- ☐ Step stools
- ☐ Bathroom steps chart
- ☐ Night light
- ☐ Indoor activities
- ☐ Cleaning supplies

Chapter 6: Getting a Little Bum on a Big Toilet

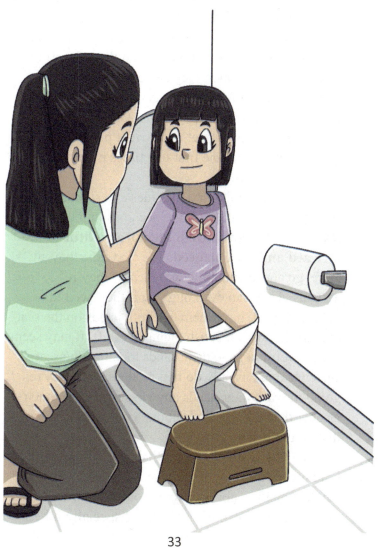

Can little bums sit on a big toilet? Yes, they can! This will, of course, look a little different than when we, as adults, sit on the toilet.

Some kids will need a step stool to help them get up on the toilet. Have them pull up their shirt a little so it's out of the way. Then, have them pull their pants all the way down to their ankles, or even all the way off, before attempting to get on the toilet. If the toilet is near a cabinet, they can use the cabinet to help support them while they get on. They could also use the wall to help support them. Once they're on, have them shimmy to get to the right position. You can help them a lot the first few times by just putting them on the toilet.

Help them hold onto the sides and sit back far enough on the seat, so all the pee goes into the toilet (especially for boys). **Help them lean a little forward and get balanced.** The first time they sit there, go ahead and hold onto them if they're nervous. They can even hug you if they need to.

To get off, have them use both hands on the seat to help shimmy and push themselves off. It may seem a little weird to have their hands touching the seat since we don't usually do that as adults, but they're going to wash their hands anyways (this is so much cleaner than having to clean out a potty chair…now that would just be gross).

If a boy is small enough that he really needs to hold onto the seat with both hands, then he's also small enough to not need to use one of his hands to point himself down while peeing. Especially if he's

Chapter 6: Getting a Little Bum on a Big Toilet

far enough back on the seat and leaning forward. After only a few times, however, he should be able to balance just fine, and it'll be no problem for him to use one of his hands to point himself down while sitting on the seat.

I recommend boys start out learning to sit on the toilet versus standing up and peeing. Sitting gives the boy more opportunities to poop. Pooping in the toilet can be a challenge, so the more opportunities the better. It's also hard for little boys to aim. Teaching them to stand and aim should be done at a later time, when they've already mastered the other bathroom steps.

I don't encourage long sitting on the toilet, waiting to pee. Especially while they're learning to balance on it. So, if they're not peeing, go ahead and take them off. Have them get back on when they're ready.

Chapter 7: Here We Go! I'll Take You Step-by-Step

The day has arrived! Just like the pros, you've already done your pre-assessment, and all your supplies are ready. You've read the chapter on the real goal, and how to be a great coach. You've set aside a couple of days, free from distractions and screens, and you're ready to go!

Go ahead and get through your morning routine before you start. Eat breakfast, get dressed, and get ready for the day. Hang up the bathroom steps chart on the wall next to the toilet, set out all your supplies, and take a deep breath because you've got this!

Steps to Teaching Potty Training

1. Teach and Model
2. Motivate
3. Help a lot!
4. Problem Solve

Step #1 Teach and Model

Make sure everyone is calm and ready when you start. This is where the teddy bear comes into play. We'll apply Play-Based Learning, in which we're going to use the teddy bear, with underwear, to model what the new expectation is.

It's important your child understands what you're trying to do and what is expected of them. It's also good that they want to do it themselves. If your child doesn't see the whole process and get what you're trying to do, then there will be some confusion, causing resistance on their end. There will also be some frustration on your part. This frustration often leads to trying to force them to sit on the toilet, and trying to force them to pee. However, modeling the expectation first will help avoid frustration.

In order for a child to learn, they need to feel safe. Make sure your tone, facial expressions, and attitude help facilitate the overall feeling of security, calm, and fun. This isn't, however, silly, goofing-off time. This process is planned and guided, but still fun. If your child thinks the teddy bear is silly, then that's ok. Just keep on going, making sure they're paying attention to your teaching. Starting with a teddy bear is not asking the child to do anything yet. They just need to fully observe and take in the information. At this moment, you're just teaching the process, expectations, and new rules.

Chapter 7: Here We Go! I'll Take You Step-by-Step

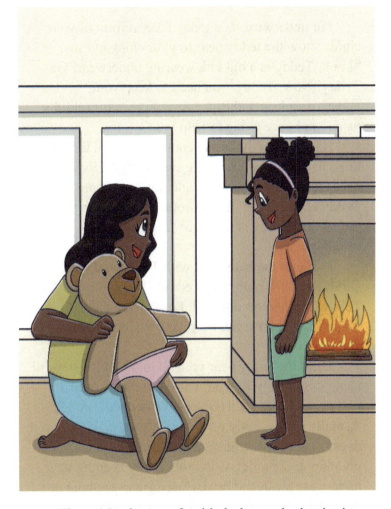

These 15 minutes of guided play at the beginning of the training is what it's going to take to show them the new expectation, which is extremely important. Having your child understand from the beginning is so worth only 15 minutes!

Put underwear on a teddy bear in front of your child. Show the teddy bear to your child and say, "Look, Teddy is a big kid, wearing underwear! Go Teddy! Now, Teddy, you need to keep your underwear clean and dry. _____ (child's name) and I are going to help you!"

Have the teddy bear pretend to tell you they need to go to the bathroom. Make sure Teddy *tells you* it needs to use the bathroom, and not *you asking* if Teddy needs to use the bathroom. We're trying to model that Teddy is taking over the hygiene responsibility.

Run into the bathroom with Teddy and your child. Say, "I'll help you, Teddy!" Show the child and Teddy the chart on the wall. Point to the chart, "Look Teddy, this is how you keep your underwear clean and dry!"

Have the teddy bear pretend to do all the steps of using the toilet, with your child watching. Actually pull down Teddy's underwear. Your child can help. Actually sit the teddy on the toilet seat, making sure it doesn't get wet of course. Say, "Teddy is peeing and pooping in the toilet. Good job Teddy keeping your underwear clean and dry by peeing and pooping in the toilet!" Wipe the teddy bear, and put the "used" toilet paper in the toilet bowl. Get Teddy off of the seat, and pull up Teddy's underwear.

Chapter 7: Here We Go! I'll Take You Step-by-Step

It's important to actually flush the toilet, so the loud sound can be associated with something positive and not something scary. Just pretend to wash Teddy's hands. No need to actually get it wet.

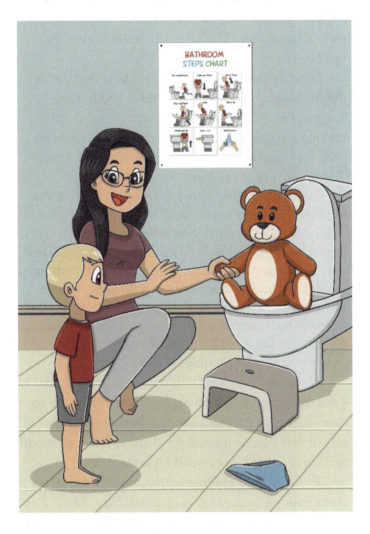

Step #2 Motivate

Having gained the child's attention with the teddy bear and showing that we're having fun together will already be a little motivating. You should have your child's full attention during the teaching time.

Point to the chart on the wall. Show that Teddy did all the steps on the chart. Praise Teddy for keeping his underwear clean and dry. Then, while making a big deal out of it, maybe even a drumroll, give the teddy bear some actual small treats. Have Teddy pretend to eat them.

See if your child asks for a treat as well. If yes, tell them they can have a treat too, if they do what Teddy did! Let's go get into underwear like Teddy! If they'd like to do what Teddy did, they can get a treat too! If they say no, and are really resistant, then finish the demonstration, and do the whole thing again a little while later. You can guide them into it, but this needs to be something they want and are motivated to do. Having the child's buy-in, or want to get a treat too, will make the training so much easier.

If the child is okay with doing what Teddy did to get a treat, then put them in underwear. It's ok to coax them a little to get them excited. It might be easier if, on the first day, you just have them in underwear with no shorts or anything over their underwear.

Praise your child for wearing underwear. Show them Teddy's underwear is clean and dry. See if their underwear is clean and dry. They should be since you just put them on. Give them a reward for having clean and dry underwear. It's their first success! Let your child know they need to keep their underwear clean and dry. They can get more treats if they pee and poop in the toilet and if they keep their underwear clean and dry. Tell them you're there to help. Let them know they need to tell you when they need to go, or if the pee starts to come, and you'll help them make it to the bathroom.

Step #3 Helping A Lot!

You'll need to really watch your child for signs that they need to pee. Every child will be a little different. This is going to take a lot of paying attention on your part. Really watch them, and try to help them recognize when they need to pee. Some children pause, try to hide, dance, pace, wiggle extra, shuffle their legs together, or touch their underwear or crotch.

If you can see they're uncomfortable, but they're not telling you they need to go, then this is the chance for you to guide them into it. They may not recognize being uncomfortable as needing to use the bathroom. You can let them know they're dancing, wiggling, or uncomfortable because they need to go to the bathroom. Remind them to tell you if they feel the pee coming, then gently help them into the bathroom. This is where the scaffolding assistance is being set up. The first few times, you really want to help them be successful.

Using the bathroom correctly is not something the child can do on their own yet, but with a more knowledgeable adult helping them, they will soon be able to. They'll need a lot of help at first in order to make it on their own. If you need to assist with the whole process for them at first, then that's okay. Pull down their underwear, get them on the seat, wipe them, etc. During the first few times of using the bathroom, you'll be building up the scaffolding, meaning you'll start with helping them a lot, and each time they go after that, you'll help with less and less.

If, while you're playing with them, you know they need to go, then help them tell you. Say, "Tell me you need to go; say, 'Mom, I need to go to the bathroom.'" If you're going to use just one word, you can say, "When you feel the pee coming, say, 'Pee Mom, pee.'" Then actually rush them into the bathroom. Help them at first with any steps they need help with. Help them be successful. As time goes on, you adjust what you help with to match their abilities. Praise them for being able to do things on their own.

Help them see the chart on the wall. Let them know that pretty soon, they'll be able to do all the steps on their own. Make this accomplishment exciting. Point out any steps they already know how to do on their own. For example, "Look, you already know how to pull down your pants and flush on your own. Pretty soon, you'll be able to do all the steps all by yourself!" You can also encourage them to try some of the steps on their own. For example, "This time, you get to try wiping on your own. I'll just be here if you need help, but I think you've got it!" Be very observant. See if they're having a hard time using the stool, and if so, why. See if they're having a hard time ripping off the toilet paper, and coach them through it. Give suggestions to them that will make each step easier.

If, after the first hour, the child hasn't needed to pee, you can give them some extra drinks to help with the process. Make sure, though, if you have them drink a lot, that you're ready to help a lot! You can offer them more drinks in the morning, then taper off before naps, and really limit the fluids before bed. I don't recommend forcing tons of drinks on them. If they end up spending all day in the bathroom, both you and the child will get burned out, and the second day will be that much harder.

Keep the treats out visible. If the child asks for a treat, then let them know they can have one if they want to go through the bathroom steps. Guide them through the steps, and then give them a treat. Remember, they don't actually have to pee or poop every time they go through the steps. If they've sat for a minute and didn't need to go, then go ahead and move them on to the remaining steps.

We're not going to be constantly asking them if they need to use the bathroom. We want *them* to take over the responsibility for their hygiene needs. We need them to feel they are in charge. Here are some things you can say:

Success With Potty Training

1. Regular reminder: "Let me know if you need to use the bathroom."
2. If you think your child *may* need to go: "I'm here to help if you need to use the bathroom. Tell me if you feel the pee coming."
3. If you see your child looking like they need to go: "Would you like me to help you use the bathroom? Let's go, I'll help you."

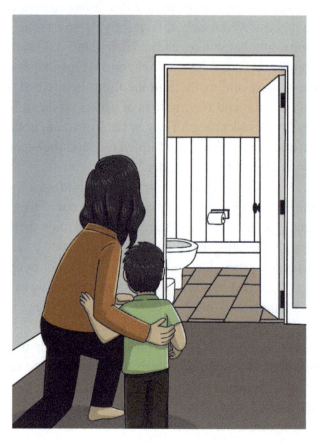

4. If it seems urgent: Pick them up, or guide them to the bathroom. "I'm going to help you keep your underwear clean and dry. Come on, let's go! You've got this! I'll help you!"

Remember to keep your tone positive. You're the positive, inspiring coach.

Reinforce that they get a reward every time they keep their underwear clean and dry. Make sure they know how to tell you if they need to go. Coach them by saying, "You say, 'Mom, I need to go to the bathroom.'" If they're nonverbal, say, "Tug on my shirt and point to your crotch." Model it for them, or have Teddy model it for them.

It's essential to give your child your full attention for at least the first day. You can't watch a show or be on your phone. You'll need to play with your child the whole time, paying close attention to what your child is doing and the signals they're giving.

Modeling Again for What to Do When They're Playing

It's good to model and role-play more than once. It gives you a chance to show what to do in different situations, and repetition is also very good for young children.

While playing with your child and Teddy, have Teddy tell you it needs to use the bathroom again. Stop what you're doing and run to the bathroom. This will model for them what needs to happen when they're playing; they'll need to stop for a minute and go to the bathroom. Praise Teddy for stopping playing and coming in to use the bathroom. Start the steps. If the child interrupts and wants to try, then go for it. If not, do all the steps with teddy, give Teddy a treat for stopping what it's doing, and keeping its underwear clean and dry.

After giving Teddy a treat, ask if your child wants a treat too. If yes, then guide them through the steps. They do not need to actually pee or poop this first time of role-playing. If they've sat for a little bit, then go ahead with the remaining steps. When done, have them notice their underwear. Say, "Yay! Your underwear is clean and dry! You get a prize!" Give them a reward.

If they do actually pee or poop in the toilet, then make sure to make a big deal out of it, with extra praise and an extra treat. Reinforce that they get a prize (or treat) every time they keep their underwear clean and dry by peeing in the toilet.

For the first couple of days, celebrate with tons of praise and maybe even a dance every time they pee or poop in the toilet. This will reinforce the good behavior. Make sure they understand you're very happy they're doing this.

Chapter 7: Here We Go! I'll Take You Step-by-Step

BATHROOM STEPS CHART ©Beth Allen

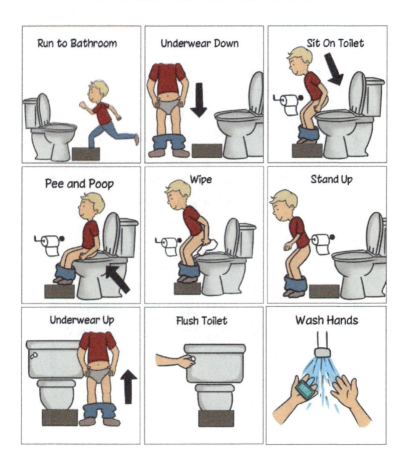

To cut out a copy of this chart, see the References at the end of the book.

Lev Vygotsky's Scaffolding

- **Getting Ready**: Gaining and maintaining the learner's interest in the task.
- **Show Me How:** Demonstrating the task.
- **Help Me Do It:** Making the task simple. Getting down on their level.
- **Controlling the Child's Level of Frustration:** Looking for triggers
- **Let Me Do It Myself:** Emphasizing certain aspects that will help with the solution.

Chapter 8: Step #4 Problem Solve

The Three Types of Problems

The number one reason parents struggle with potty training is that variables come up that the parent doesn't know how to handle. Usually, parents stop potty training because they get confused about what to do, not because the child isn't ready. I have found there are three types of problems that come up: *understanding*, *motivational*, and *behavioral*. Before I jump into these problems, I want to remind you that this is your precious child. You love them! You want them to succeed, and they need *you* in order to do it.

> **Three Types of Problems**
> - Understanding
> - Motivational
> - Behavioral

Problem #1: Understanding

It's important to assess where your child is in the process. Ask yourself if your child seems to understand each part of the process, or if your child seems to be stuck on one of the steps.

Success With Potty Training

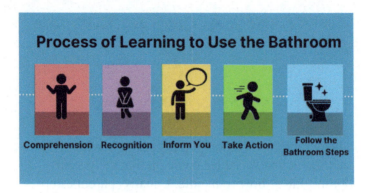

Here's the process of learning to use the bathroom:

1. **Comprehension**: Your child understands what you're trying to do.
2. **Recognition**: Your child can recognize when they need to pee or poop.
3. **Inform You**: Your child tells you they need to go.
4. **Take Action:** Once your child recognizes they need to go, they need to start into action.
5. **Follow the Bathroom Steps:** Once in action, they need to follow the bathroom steps on the chart.

Here's what to do if they're having trouble with one of the steps:

1. **Comprehension**: Model and role-play again with the teddy bear. (See Chapter 7)

2. **Recognition**: Look for cues of when they need to go. Really watch and pay attention. When you see your child acting uncomfortable, or holding themselves, or fidgeting, etc., point it out to them. Tell them, "What you're feeling is the pee coming. When the pee comes, it's time to go to the bathroom!" Then quickly take them in. Some examples of cues are:
    a. Holding or touching their crotch or bum
    b. Stopping what they're doing and holding still
    c. Fidgeting
    d. Pacing or dancing
    e. Wiggling their legs
    f. Stressed look on their face
    g. Hiding somewhere

3. **Inform You**: Once you've pointed out it's time to use the bathroom, rush them to the bathroom, and tell them what to say. For instance, "When the pee comes, you say 'Mom, pee!'" Keep repeating what you want them to say *as you're taking them*. "Mom, pee, pee!" When they do say or do something to tell you, make sure to pay attention to it and give them a reward for it. For example, "You tugged on my shirt to let me know you needed to go to the bathroom; you get a sticker!" Do a lot of reflection after an accident. What did

you see them doing beforehand? Was there anything that might have been a cue?

4. **Take Action**: After seeing their cue, let them know it's time to go! Move them into action. Role-playing this again when it's not an emergency will help. Explain that when you're in the playroom, and you feel pee coming, you need to use your fast feet. "Let's see your fast feet go! Show me! Ready, set, go!" Run into the bathroom. "Let's see how fast you are at getting up out of bed if you need to go. Okay, lay down and then show me your fast feet. Ready, Set, Go! Wow, you're so fast!" Make it a game to practice running in. You can race them, or have teddy race them. Tell them that when the pee is coming, we need to stop what we're doing and then we need fast, racing feet to go quickly to the bathroom.

5. **Follow the Bathroom Steps:** This is where a lot of the scaffolding takes place. Go ahead and assist them toward success. At first, you may need to pull down their underwear and put them on the toilet, so they can be successful and not have an accident. Look at each step on the chart, and take note of the step(s) they're having trouble with. What instructions would help them? Be kind, patient, and helpful. Adjust your assistance to fit how they're doing. If they need more help,

then help them more. If they're trying to do it on their own, offer less help. Watch for their level of frustration. Too much frustration isn't good. A little frustration is okay.

Problem #2: Motivational

My child just doesn't want to do this!

This is a great time to do a quick self-assessment. How stressed are you by this? How much patience do you have right now? Are you projecting your stress onto your child? A child doesn't want to be part of a stressful situation. Are you smiling and being kind? Was the modeling fun? Did you capture their attention? Were you showing excitement?

Take a look at your treasure box. Do you have rewards that are truly motivating your child? Do you need to mix it up? You can also place the rewards in a place easily seen as a reminder of what they earn when they use the bathroom.

Progress Charts:

To help motivate, I like to use progress charts. See the Reference section for an example chart. These are just like sticker charts, but it doesn't need to be an official chart. You can have any old paper, or you can just use their shirt. The nice part about stickers is that they aren't eaten, so you can refer back to them and remind them of all the good progress they've made.

Here's how it works: you give them a sticker every time they do something you want them to be working on. This is just another motivator. For instance, I would show them the stickers and say, "Look at all these awesome stickers! I want to give you one of these when you tell Mommy that you need to go. I'm so excited to give you one, once you tell Mommy you need to use the bathroom." Then, when they do tell you, and you get through the bathroom process, you give them a treat for peeing, and a sticker for telling you they needed to go.

Later on, you point out the sticker again. "Wow, you got that one for telling me you needed to go to the bathroom. Good job! I have more stickers I'd love to give you for when you tell me when the pee is coming. You'll get so many stickers! Your paper will look so good!"

Change up what you give the sticker for. Try to move their progression forward. Figure out what you want to focus on, and use the sticker for that. I've found progress charts work really well for older children who need extra motivation.

Problem #3: Behavioral

What we're asking our children to do when potty training, is to change their behavior. We're not just asking them to learn something new. So, although we may have taught it well, changing their behavior is taking it to another level.

I think back to when I was on my last diet. I learned a lot, and I was successful. I lost some weight, which was great. So why then did I find myself dieting again a few months later? Well, with every change of behavior, there is a maintenance period and a relapse. You can take action and be successful, but then you must *maintain* it. Psychologists have studied this for years. Two psychologists in particular, Prochaska and DiClemente, have coined this as "The Cycle of Change."[7]

It's going to be very important for you and any other caregiver to help maintain the new expectation. The child will get tired and want to go back to old ways, but you can't let them! If you need to, continue with the rewards, modeling, and scaffolding. If you give up, the child will too, and there will inevitably be a relapse.

---

[7] Ignacio Pacheco, "The Cycle of Change," Social Work Tech, January 9, 2012, http://socialworktech.com/2012/01/09/stages-of-change-prochaska-diclemente/

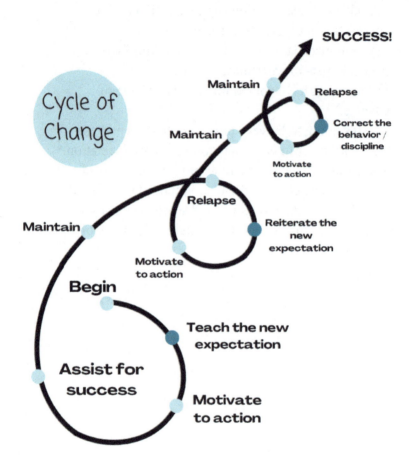

Relapse

If a child goes into relapse, then you'll need to help them get back on track. You'll need to help them be aware that this relapse is a problem. Correct the behavior. Remind them of what is expected of them. Help them get motivated again into action. Then be more diligent with the maintenance period.

For example, if my child was potty trained but then a few days later went behind the couch and peed, I would take my child to the accident, point to it, and tell them, "Pee does not go behind the couch, pee goes in the toilet. It is not ok to pee anywhere else." I would then take my child to the bathroom. I would point to the chart and to the toilet and say, "This is where the pee goes. You need to tell me when you need to go, and I can help you if you need. You need to stop what you're doing, and run into the bathroom and pee here, in the toilet." I would then remind them that they don't get rewards for peeing behind the couch. I would then reinstate the rewards, and let them know that they can have a sticker when they pee in the toilet, but, they can't have a sticker now, because they didn't pee in the right place.

If the child is older, I would then say, "I have to clean up the pee. You'll have to help me." If the child is defiant or if I really don't want them cleaning the pee or poop, then I could say, "I have to clean up the pee; you'll have to sit in time out while I clean up the pee. We both have to stop what we were doing until this mess gets cleaned up."

If the child has been successful with potty training for some while and then just stops, then you treat this as you would any other behavioral problem. If you're not sure, you can ask yourself, "What would I do if they had colored on the wall? What would I do if they had purposefully thrown all their food across the kitchen?" If you don't currently have a system for handling situations like this, then now is a great time to start. Time-outs are great. There are loads of books that can help you get a system in place. I like the book *1-2-3 Magic* by Thomas W. Phelan.

You are in charge of your home, not your child. You can calmly and sternly reinforce the rules. Peeing and pooping only in the toilet *is* one of the rules of the home.

Changing behavior isn't perfect. We don't, as human beings, go in a straight line of progression. Prochaska and DiClemente describe it more as an upward spiral. We may relapse, but we learn from each relapse. Hopefully, each relapse becomes smaller and shorter as we continually get back on track towards the goal.

★★★

For the first couple of days and nights, you will really need to take some time to pay attention. As you pay close attention and problem solve, ask yourself, "Is this an understanding problem, a motivational problem, or a behavioral problem?"

When something is going wrong, take a moment, and get *curious* instead of getting mad or frustrated. Being a curious detective will go so much further toward solving the problem than being mad or frustrated.

Chapter 9: Accidents

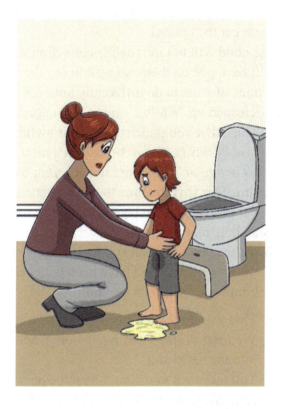

Accidents will happen, and are an important part of the process. If your child pees or poops in their underwear or on the floor, have them go into (or carry them into) the bathroom. Have them take their underwear off. Tell them, "Oh, no, your underwear isn't clean and dry." Remind them you're here to help them, if they'll let you know when they need to go to the bathroom. You're here to help them keep their underwear clean and dry. If they tell you when the pee is coming, you'll help them get to the toilet on time. We only pee and poop in the toilet. This will help them get the reward.

The child will not internalize correction while they still have pee on them, so wait to say the instructions of what to do differently until *after* your child is cleaned up. While cleaning them up, acknowledge that you understand this is awful. *Point out how yucky this is, and acknowledge that it feels gross and not good.* Make sure to keep your tone of voice calm. This isn't the time to be energetic or happy, but it is the time to be empathetic, understanding, and reinforcing.

When the child is clean and feels safe again, give instructions on what should have been done. Here are some examples of what can be said:

- That was awful getting all yucky, wasn't it?
- We need to stop what we're doing, and run into the bathroom.
- Tell me when you start to feel the pee coming.
- Run fast to the bathroom when you feel the pee coming.
- Tell Mom when you need to go, so I can help you.
- Don't wait to go to the bathroom.
- Go to the bathroom right away, really fast.
- Remember, you need to keep your underwear clean and dry, so you don't get all yucky.
- I'm here to help you.

Clean up the child and the mess. Do not give out rewards for accidents. Let them know they missed the opportunity for the reward, but they can get a reward next time if they keep their underwear clean and dry.

Accidents will happen and are an important part of the process. The reason I don't encourage padded training pants, padded underwear, or pull-ups is that accidents need to be something the child hates, not something that feels the same as it did before. When pee or poop runs down their legs and gets them all gross, it will be a new, awful experience. It's important to stay calm and in coach mode when an accident happens. Remember, you're outside the boxing ring, coaching your child what they can do differently.

Great coaches do a review of the game. They try hard to learn from previous mistakes. After each accident, it's good to do a review. Be the detective and figure out why the accident happened, so you can coach your child through not having another one. Do a lot of reflection after an accident.

You can ask these questions:

- What did I see them doing beforehand?
- Was there anything that might have been a clue that they needed to go?
- Why did this happen?
- What was the child doing? (Distracted by a screen? Didn't know how to pause?)
- What was I doing? Was I distracted?

- What were the obstacles? (Hard to pull down pants, didn't know where the bathroom was in a new place?)
- Was this an understanding, motivational, or behavioral problem?

Once you figure out what went wrong, role-play with your child what to do next time. For instance, if your child was playing and didn't stop to pee, then you could have your child start in the playroom and race you to the bathroom. You can say, "Here we are in the playroom, but if we need to use the bathroom, we should run to the bathroom. Let's practice. Ready, set, go! Run to the bathroom!"

Chapter 10: Training for Naps and Night

Naps and Nighttime

I like to potty train for naps and nighttime at the same time I potty train during the day. I really want to show consistency with the child. This will be up to you, though between the ages of two and four and a half, the size of the bladder doubles. A child who's just 22 months may not be able to go a whole night without peeing. But, by the time they're four and a half, they shouldn't have a problem. I have found by the time a child is 30 months old, they are just fine going the night without peeing. How old your child is will help you decide what's best. Start off training for naps. A two-year-old can easily go two hours between peeing. Having your child dry for naps will help you gain your confidence for night training.

Purchase a waterproof mattress protector in advance and have it already on the mattress. Make sure the child can get out of their bed if they need to use the bathroom. They cannot be confined in a crib or gated room.

The steps for teaching and modeling are the same for bedtime and naps as during the day. If getting your child to sleep is a struggle, then do the teddy bear modeling at an earlier time of day.

Before putting your child down, have them use the bathroom. Do not put them down with a bottle or sippy cup. Liquids should be limited after dinner time. This will help your child be successful. Your child may have a small drink before bed but definitely should not be going to bed with a drink in hand. If you've been using a cup as a soothing tool for your child to sleep, consider replacing it with reading them a book or singing them a lullaby.

We will use the teddy bear again to show the new rules and expectations. We need to show the child what to do and how to do it. Have Teddy lie down in the child's bed. Emphasize that Teddy is clean and dry. Pat the bed and teach that while Teddy is sleeping, he needs to not only stay clean and dry but also keep the *bed* clean and dry. Then have Teddy need to go to the bathroom. Show Teddy getting up and going into the bathroom to pee.

Make sure to actually walk down the hall to where the bathroom is, so the child learns the path from the bedroom to the bathroom. Explain that Teddy is doing a great job keeping his underwear, pants, *and bed* clean and dry. Let your child know that if they keep their bed clean and dry, they'll get a treat when they wake up. Make sure your child knows if they need you at night, they can come to get you, and you'll be there to help.

Chapter 10: Training for Naps and Night

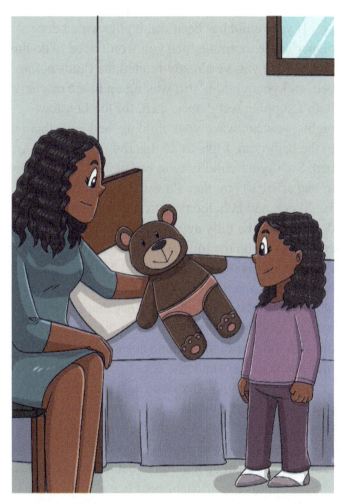

Once you have put the child to bed, there aren't any more rewards for the night. We want to encourage them to go to sleep. If they get up to pee, you can praise them for staying dry and let them know they'll get their reward in the morning when they wake up.

If your child has been waking up with a dry diaper in the morning, then you won't need to do this next part. If you've already limited the fluids before bed, and your child is still waking up in the morning with a sopping wet diaper, then, for the first few nights, you can wake your child up, and have them go to the bathroom. I like to do this right before I go to bed. So, if your child goes to bed at 7:30 pm and I go to bed at 10:30 pm, then I'd wake the child up at 10:30 pm, and help them go to the bathroom. They don't need to be fully awake for this, just awake enough to sit on the toilet. (I've been known to carry them in and set them on the toilet.) Then put them back in bed. Waking them up is not a must. If they've woken up in the morning with a dry diaper, or a barely wet diaper, then try to see if they make it through the first night with no accidents. If so, then this step doesn't need to be done.

In the morning, your child will probably need to pee right when they wake up, but they won't be used to rushing to the bathroom. Make sure to wake up *before your child*, and as soon as you hear them start to rustle, get them up and to the bathroom. This will greatly improve their chances of being successful.

Nighttime Accidents

If they have an accident during the night, remember you're still the calm, supportive coach. Take off the wet clothes, set the child on the toilet to finish, and reinforce that's where the pee goes. Quickly get them cleaned off, rinsed off in the bath if necessary, and back in bed. I have you get two mattress protectors so you can throw the wet bedding in a basket for the night, to be cleaned in the morning.

In the morning, talk to them about staying dry at night. Talk to them about getting out of bed to pee and not peeing in bed. Role-play not peeing on the bed. Have them lie on their bed and then get up and run to the bathroom. This is a great thing to do as a game during the day, when everyone is awake and alert and not trying to be put down for bed at night. When they go to bed that night, remind them of the role-playing you did earlier.

Chapter 11: It's All You Kid
Taking Down the Scaffolding

What does it mean to be trained? When are you finished?

Remember, the initial goal is that you want them to take care of their own hygiene needs, wear underwear, and keep their underwear clean and dry. It may take a while before you're not helping out at all with this process, whether it's helping sufficiently wipe after pooping, or helping find the bathroom at Grandma's. Although your child is still needing some assistance, after a couple of days, they should be able to get the process down, allowing you to venture out, and go back to your routine without many accidents.

You'll probably be giving out rewards for the next couple of weeks, but the *way* you give out these rewards will change. At the end of the weekend, look at the bathroom steps chart. Like any good teacher, do a re-assessment. What is your child able to do? What are they still working on? Adjust the treats and rewards to be earned when your child does something you want them to work on. For instance, if the child isn't wiping by themselves, you can say, "Today you get a treat if you wipe all by yourself." (Or getting on the toilet all by yourself, or pulling up your pants all by yourself, etc., whatever they're still working on.) Just make sure the changes in how they receive treats are announced *ahead of time*, so the expectations remain clear to them.

Total independence is going to take time, maybe even a few months, and that's okay and normal. If your child hasn't grasped the concept in the first couple of days, then keep re-assessing, problem-solving, modeling, and role-playing even up to 10 days. If, after 10 days, it's still not going well, it might be time to talk with your pediatrician. A pediatrician can help in seeing if there may be a medical reason why your child is having trouble.

Taking a Break

If you really can't take it anymore, it's okay to call it quits and try again another time. If you've come to this point, make sure to take some time for reflection. What went wrong? What were the biggest obstacles? Were *you* ready? How can training go better next time? Write down your thoughts and the details from your re-assessment, so you can use them next time. Then, break for at least 10 days before you try again, so you can have a fresh start.

Please take a moment to remember how *precious* your little one is. Remind yourself that you love them! You're their biggest fan, and their best teacher! They desperately need you! They need you to be fully engaged, and this is something you can do! Now take a breather, say a prayer, and know that you've got this! Parenting is hard, hard stuff, but your child needs you! You've taken on this great responsibility

Chapter 11: It's All You Kid

and teaching your child will be the most important thing you do in your life.

Taking a break is not giving up. It's just reflecting on what can be done better and what changes need to be made in order for this to be successful for both you and your child.

Chapter 12: The Scoop on Poop

If getting your child to poop in the toilet is a challenge, you're not alone. A lot of children take longer to understand the concept of now pooping in the toilet. So, here are my tips for dealing with poop.

With diapers, some children are on a poop schedule. You've come to know their schedule and it's pretty regular. A lot of children will also poop more than once a day with diapers. As soon as you start to potty train though, the schedule will go out the door. You will also notice your child will poop less often. This is all completely normal. Your child is learning to control their bowel movements and, in doing so, is creating a new routine with it. It's okay if they're not pooping every single day at first. Their body is trying to figure this out.

If your child hasn't pooped for a while, then you can do a few things to encourage it. You can have them sit a little longer on the toilet. Sit in the bathroom with them and sing, or read them a book. Encourage them to try pushing. Hug them for comfort if needed. Remember though, this is *not a punishment*, so don't force them to sit too long. Keep the mood light and calm.

One reason I have boys start out sitting on the toilet for peeing is that it gives them more opportunities to try to poop. The more opportunities they have to sit, the more opportunities there will be to try to poop.

Constipation

If your child is constipated, make sure your child is eating healthy foods. Ask yourself, is my child eating fiber? Has my child had any fresh fruits and veggies? It's also important for your child to get exercise. Pay attention if the child is the one doing the exercising. So many times, we put them in a stroller, cart, or bike carrier when we're exercising. We then think they're exercising too, when they're just spending the day sitting. Running around a living room may not be enough exercise to keep their bowel movements regular.

If you're having continued problems with pooping or constipation, then discuss options with your pediatrician.

Wiping

It's important for a child to practice wiping. I like to have the child wipe and then I'm just there for the double check. When I double check, I'll show them when there was more poop to be wiped. Let them know they need to keep wiping until there's no more poop. Remind them that they're wanting to keep their underwear clean and dry. Show them when it's clean. If their underwear has poop on it, then show them the underwear and explain that it's not clean.

Have them wipe away from the body, from the middle out. It's especially important for girls to wipe poop away from their vagina and urinary tract, so they do not get any poop in it.

Poop Accidents

Poop accidents should be treated the same as pee accidents. If your child poops in their underwear or on the floor, walk or carry them to the bathroom. Have them take their underwear off. Tell them, "Oh, no, your underwear isn't clean and dry." Remind them you're here to help them if they'll let you know when they need to go to the bathroom. You're here to help them keep their underwear clean and dry. If they tell you when the poop is coming, you'll help them get to the toilet on time. We only pee and poop in the toilet. This will help them get the reward.

Let them know that they don't get a reward when there are accidents. You can say things like, "Oh no, no treat!" or, "I'm so sorry, no treat. Your underwear is dirty. No treats for dirty underwear. Let me know next time you feel the poop coming. Run to the bathroom if the poop is coming and I'll help you so you can get a treat next time." You may feel like a broken record, but the repetition and consistency are vitally important to their success.

Take time to reflect on what happens each time there is an accident, so you can problem solve and avoid the accident in the future. See Chapter 9 on accidents and Chapter 8 on problem solving for more great tips.

Chapter 13: More Help!

First Time Out of the House

The first time you go out, bring a change of clothes for your child, including socks, a plastic bag to put wet clothes into, and wipes just in case. You can even put something plastic on their car seat that they can sit on if you're worried. (A grocery bag works well.) Do not, however, put them in a pull-up. Be brave! You've got this! When you get to where you're going, explain the expectations again. Point out the bathroom, first-thing. Remind them to tell you when they need to go, and that you'll help them.

Car Trips

Have them use the bathroom before getting into the car (a good habit, even for adults). Watch their fluids, so you can time when you need to stop. There are some great travel potties you could buy if you're going to be several hours in-between rest stops. Bring extra clothes, wipes, and sanitizing supplies, just in case.

Assess how they've been doing during the training process. If you're nervous, you can have them sit on a plastic grocery bag just in case. There are also plastic inserts that fit on car seats that are great for bigger accidents. You can also buy the bed wetting mats and have them sit on those as well.

If, after you've assessed how they've been doing, you've noted they've never been dry for their nap or at night, and you know they'll fall asleep in the car, then you can put a diaper on over their underwear for the trip. Do not leave this diaper on after you arrive at your destination.

Tips

- Lots of treats at the beginning with explanations as to why they're getting the treat works really well. For example, "Good job stopping playing and coming into the bathroom, and good job getting yourself on the toilet." Start to wean off the treats after some successful times.

- Make corrections, like a positive coach. Remind them you're there to help. They just need to let you know sooner.

- Keep the play on the same floor of the home as the bathroom. Don't bring stairs into the mix. Make sure the bathroom has easy access. No obstacles, like laundry baskets or doggy gates.

- If they seem to be bored of the treats, then change them up. Cereal pieces one day, marshmallows the next, stickers the next, etc.

Proper Wiping

Wipe away from the *front* of the body. Poop should be wiped away from the front of the body. The vagina should be wiped down towards the middle. You want to avoid ever getting poop in the vagina.

Little boys seem to dribble afterward, so teaching them to wipe usually gets the little bit that's left. Sometimes having them give the penis a little tap afterward also helps.

FAQs

What happens if it's been several nights, and my child is still peeing the bed? I'm exhausted!

The only time you might use a diaper for sleeping is if you're at your wit's end with nighttime accidents. You've already tried for several nights, and you just need to get a good night's sleep (I'm a big advocate of sleep). But be warned, if you use a diaper for sleeping, you will experience some regression in training and will have to retrain for nighttime hygiene at a later date. Ask yourself these questions when assessing nighttime accidents.

- Are they going to bed with a cup or bottle in hand?
- Am I limiting liquids after dinner?

- Is there something stopping them from getting up to use the bathroom? Are they scared?
- Have I tried waking them up at night and having them use the bathroom?
- Have I tried waking them up a few minutes earlier than they usually get up to get them to the bathroom first thing in the morning?

If you've tried everything, and it's still not working, then this would be a good time to talk things over with your pediatrician to see if there may be a medical reason why your child is having a hard time.

What happens if my child backslides?

If you start to see some back sliding, then adjust your rewards. Remind them of the chart on the wall and that they can follow the chart, so they don't miss any steps. Take a quick assessment of yourself as well. Have you let some things slide and not been consistent with the expectations? *You'll* need to be consistent in order for them to be successful. (See Chapter 8 for relapse.)

What if, after the weekend, my child is still having accidents?

If your child hasn't grasped the concept in the first couple of days, keep re-assessing, problem-solving, modeling, and role-playing even up to 10 days. If, after 10 days it's still not going well, it might be time to take a break and talk with your pediatrician. A pediatrician can help see if there may be a medical reason why your child is having trouble. (See Chapter 11 Taking a Break.)

My child was trained, but now, several weeks later, is peeing their pants.

This is a behavioral problem. Refer to Chapter 8 on problem-solving. Sometimes there are outside things happening to cause your child to digress. Ask yourself:

- Is there a new baby?
- Does your child need more attention?
- Did your child change schools?
- Are they sick?
- Did we just move?
- Do they have pinworms? Or a rash?
- Are they having added stress or nightmares?
- Did we go on vacation and get completely off our normal schedule?

If so, try to acknowledge the problem. Remind them you're here for them. Problem solve. If needed, put the chart back up, and help them through the steps again.

If a building starts to fall after it's been built, then up comes the scaffolding again until the damage has been repaired. This doesn't mean putting them back in diapers, but it means being extra alert and helpful again to get them back on track.

Chapter 14: I Have to Go to Work!

Sending Them to Their Caregiver

You've got to go back to work, so here are some tips for sending your child back to school, daycare, or other care providers.

Before Training:
- Tell the school, teacher, or daycare provider that you're planning on potty training. Get their input.
- Ask them for their potty-training guidelines or practices.
- Ask for the schedule. See if they have scheduled bathroom breaks, and if you'll need to try to train towards those.
- Ask how they respond to accidents.

During Training:
- Pay close attention to how your child is doing and how they respond to different situations, such as accidents.
- Compare and contrast what you're doing to how the school will do it.
- If your school has scheduled bathroom breaks, keep track of when your child is peeing and compare that to the breaks.

- Make adaptations as needed so the adjustment to the caregiver setting will be a success.

After Training:
- Talk with your caregiver. Let them know how it went.
- At drop-off, show your child the toilet, in relation to their normal classroom or play space.
- Remind your child of the new expectations.
- Let your child know who to tell if they need to go.
- Make sure to drop off a couple of changes of clothes with them.
- Provide the caregiver with the same rewards system you had. For example, if you used a sticker chart for progress, you can drop off the chart and stickers.
- Provide the necessary precautions for naptime.

A Small Ask

Now that you finished reading this book, what did you think of what you read? Were there any tips or information you found insightful? What do you think was missing from this book? While you're thinking back on what you read, it'll mean the world to me if you left an honest review on Amazon.

As you know, reviews play an integral part in building relevancy for books. So, whether you found the information helpful or not, your candid review will help other customers make an informed purchase.

Also, based on your review, I'll adjust future editions. This way, we can all learn and grow.

Thank you!

Success With Potty Training

Plan Outline

Start Date_____.

I have cleared my schedule.

For my other kids I have _____ taking care of them.

I have my supplies. (See Chapter 5 for supplies.)

    My indoor activities to do with my child that *aren't on a screen* are:

    _____.

    My treasure box of rewards includes:

    _____
    _____.

What I'm going to do:

    Teach and model.
    Motivate.
    Watch for cues and help my child recognize cues.
    Help my child to success.
    Problem Solve.

When my child has an accident, I will_____.
(See Chapter 9 on accidents.)

When my child throws a tantrum, I will_____.
(See Chapter 8 on the three types of problems.)

When I lose my patience, I will
_____.

(Take five minutes in my room. Eat chocolate. Deep breath. Call and vent to my mom. Remember you're on the same team. Remember this is your precious child, whom you love. You're the coach, there to help your child accomplish something great!)

BATHROOM STEPS CHART ©Beth Allen

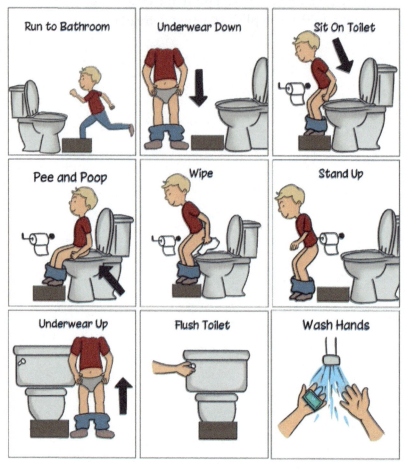

Cut out this chart from References in the back of the book. Go to www.successwithpottytraining.com to download a full-page chart.

To empower is to believe your child is capable of becoming more than they think they can, and then lovingly help them accomplish more.

About the Author

Beth Allen has a passion for helping young moms succeed. Getting your feet underneath you as a mom can be challenging, and Beth wants to empower moms and help them realize they can do this! Beth is a mom of four and is a Certified Potty Training Consultant with the Institute of Pediatric Sleep and Parenting. She has her Bachelor's degree from Brigham Young University.

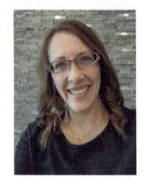

Index

A

Accidents, **59**, **63**, **79**
    night time, **70**
    poop, **79**
Assessments
    eighth bladder control, **25**
    eleventh health, **26**
    fifth no crib, **24**
    first communicating their needs, **21**
    fourth pulling down and up pants, **22**
    ninth walking and climbing, **25**
    second following simple instructions, **21**
    seventh diapers are yucky, **24**
    sixth no drink in bed, **24**
    tenth your child's understanding, **25**
    third sitting independently, **24**
    twelfth fears, **26**

B

Back sliding, **84**
Bathroom steps chart, **32**, **37**, **40**, **44**, **54**, **73**
Behavior, **56**
Behavioral problem, **56**, **60**, **61**, **84**
Bladder control, **25**
Boxing ring, **10**, **65**

C

Car seat, **81**
Car trips, **81**
Child development, **12**, **17**
Childcare provider, **87**
Clean and dry, **42**
Cleaning supplies, **32**
Climbing, **25**
Coach, **7**, **10**, **13**
Communicating, **25**
Comprehension, **51**, **52**
Constipation, **78**
Crib, **24**
Cycle of Change, **57**, **58**

D

Daycare, **87**
Determined child, **16**
Diaper, **24**, **70**
    dry at night, **27**
DiClemente, **57**, **60**
Drink, **24**
Drinks, **45**

E

Erik Erikson, **12**
Expectations, **38**, **39**, **68**

F

Fears, **26**
Flushing, **41**
Focused child, **15**
Follow the bathroom steps, **52**, **54**
Frequently asked questions, **83**

G

Goal, **7, 8, 9,** 73
   the right goal, **7**
   the wrong, **7**
Guided play, **39**

H

Health, **26**
Help them be successful, **44**

I

Indoor activities, **32**
Inform you, **52, 53**

L

Lev Vygotsky, **17**
   scaffolding, **17**

M

Maintenance, **57, 59**
Mattress protector, **31**
Model, **52**
Modeling, **15, 19, 40**
   while playing, **47**
Morning, **70, 71**
Motivated child, **15**
Motivational problem, **55, 61**
   progress chart, **55**

N

Naps and night time, **67**
Night time, **67**
   accidents, **70, 83**
Nightlight, **32**

P

Padded training pants, **65**
Padded underwear, **65**
Persistent child, **15**
Plan outline, **89, 101**
Play-based learning, **3, 15, 19, 37**
Playing, **47**
Poop, **77**
   accidents, **79**
   holding it, **77**
   schedule, **77**
   wiping, **78**
Potty chairs, **31**
Problem solving, **51, 61**
Process of potty training, **52**
   follow the bathroom steps, **52**
   inform you, **52**
   recognition, **52**
   take action, **52**
   understanding, **52**
Processof Learning to Use the Bathroom. *See* Process of potty training
Prochaska, **57, 60**
Progress charts, **55**
Progression, **56**
Pull down pants, **23**
Pull up pants, **23**
Pull-ups, **65, 83**

Q

Quitting, **74**

R

Recognition, **52, 53**

Index

Recognizing they need to pee, **43**
Relapse, **59**
Reminders, **43**, **46**
Reward, **69**, **73**, *See* Treat
   when not to give, **59**, **65**
Rewards, **9**, **31**
Role-play, **52**, **54**, **66**
   night time, **71**

S

Scaffolding, **17**, **19**, **43**, **54**
   taking down, **73**
School, **87**
Signs they need to pee, **43**
Sitting independently, **24**
Step #1 Teach and Model, **37**
Step#2 Motivate, **42**
Step#3 Helping a Lot, **43**
Step#4 Problem Solve, **51**
Stool, **32**
Supplies, **31**

T

Take action, **52**, **54**

Taking a break, **74**
Teddy bear, **37**, **39**, **40**, **68**
   playing, **47**
Three types of problems, **51**
Time-out, **60**
Tips, **82**
Toilet, **8**, **34**
Training pants, **65**
Treasure box, **31**
Treat, **31**, **42**, **45**, **48**

U

Uncomfortable, **43**
Understanding, **51**, **52**
Understanding problem, **51**, **61**
Underwear, **8**, **42**
   clean and dry, **8**, **40**, **42**, **48**

W

Washing hands, **41**
Waterproof mattress protector, **31**
Wiping, **82**
   poop, **78**
Work, **87**

References

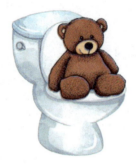

Process of Learning to Use the Bathroom

Comprehension	Recognition	Inform You	Take Action	Follow the Bathroom Steps
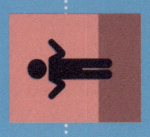	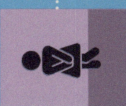	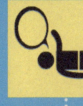		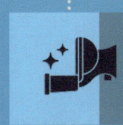

Success With Potty Training

Plan Outline

Start Date_____.

I have cleared my schedule.

For my other kids I have _____ taking care of them.

I have my supplies. (See Chapter 5 for supplies.)

> My indoor activities to do with my child that *aren't on a screen* are:
> _____.
>
> My treasure box of rewards includes:
> _____
> _____.

What I'm going to do:

> Teach and model.
> Motivate.
> Watch for cues and help my child recognize cues.
> Help my child to success.
> Problem Solve.

When my child has an accident, I will_____.
(See Chapter 9 on accidents.)

When my child throws a tantrum, I will_____.
(See Chapter 8 on the three types of problems.)

When I lose my patience, I will
_____.
(Take five minutes in my room. Eat chocolate. Deep breath. Call and vent to my mom. Remember you're on the same team. Remember this is your precious child, whom you love. You're the coach, there to help your child accomplish something great!)

Supplies Quick List

See Chapter 5 for more details.

- ☐ Underwear
- ☐ Easy clothes
- ☐ Teddy bear
- ☐ Treats or rewards (treasure box)
- ☐ Waterproof mattress protectors (2)
- ☐ Step stools
- ☐ Bathroom steps chart
- ☐ Night light
- ☐ Indoor activities
- ☐ Cleaning supplies

Success With Potty Training

Pre-Assessment Checklist

See Chapter 4 for more details.

My Child:
- ☐ Communicates their needs
- ☐ Follows simple instructions
- ☐ Sits independently
- ☐ Can pull down and up pants
- ☐ No crib or confined bedroom situation
- ☐ Weaned off any liquids in bed
- ☐ Has been prepped that diapers are yucky
- ☐ Has dry spells in-between dirty diapers
- ☐ Can walk and climb
- ☐ My child communicates they understand me by _____.
- ☐ My child communicates they don't understand me by _____.
- ☐ In good health
- ☐ I have addressed Fears

Success With Potty Training

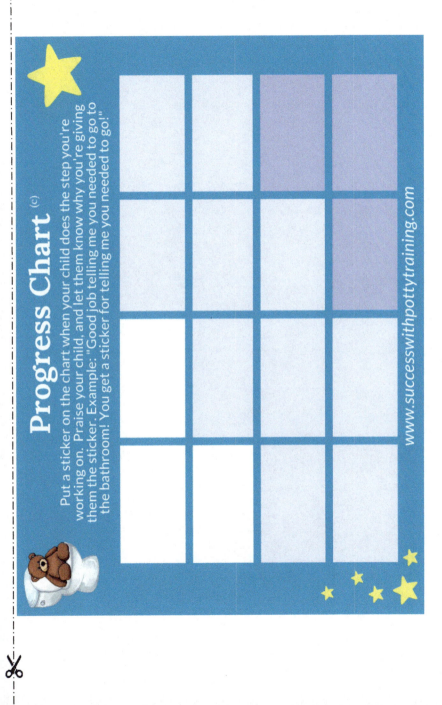

Success With Potty Training

Loved the book? Leave a review on Amazon!

BATHROOM STEPS CHART ©Beth Allen

Run to Bathroom	Underwear Down	Sit On Toilet
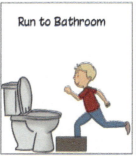	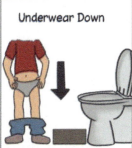	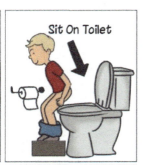
Pee and Poop	**Wipe**	**Stand Up**
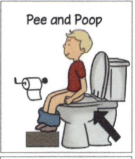	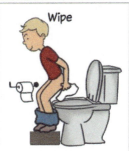	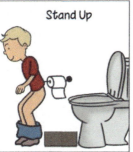
Underwear Up	**Flush Toilet**	**Wash Hands**
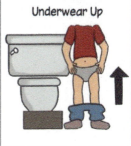	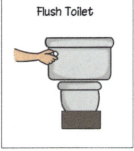	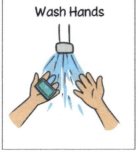

 You can download a full-page copy at www.successwithpottytraining.com.

Made in the USA
Las Vegas, NV
12 April 2024